The Secrets To Eternal Youth

Uncovering the Hidden Path To Living Your Longest, Healthiest Life

BY 

DR. KATE WINFREY

<u>Disclaimer:</u>

The information presented in "The Secrets to Eternal Youth: Uncovering the Hidden Path To Living Your Longest, Healthiest Life" is for educational and informational purposes only.
The author of this book is not a licensed medical professional and the information contained herein is not intended to be a substitute for professional medical advice, diagnosis, or treatment.

The author has made every effort to ensure that the information provided in this book is accurate and up-to-date.
However, the author and publisher do not accept any responsibility for any loss, damage, or injury arising from the use of the information presented in this book.

Readers are encouraged to seek the advice of a licensed medical professional before making any changes to their diet, exercise routine, or lifestyle. The author and publisher shall not be held liable for any direct or indirect damages arising from the use of the information provided in this book.

The information presented in this book is based on the author's personal experience and research. Results may vary based on individual circumstances,
and the author and publisher make no guarantees as to the effectiveness or safety of any of the recommendations contained herein.

By reading this book, you acknowledge that you have read and understood this disclaimer and agree to hold the author and publisher harmless from any and all claims or damages arising from your use of the information presented herein.

Thank You

Table Of Contents

Table Of Contents .... - 3 -

Introduction .... - 5 -

Chapter 1 .... - 8 -

The Science of Aging

Chapter 2 .... - 17 -

The Power of Nutrition

Chapter 3 .... - 27 -

Exercise and Movement

Chapter 4 .... - 32 -

Managing Stress and Mental Health

Chapter 5 .... - 36 -

Sleep and Rest

Chapter 6 .... - 40 -

Lifestyle Choices for Eternal Youth

Conclusion .... - 43 -

<u>Introduction</u>

As humans, we are always searching for ways to live longer and healthier lives. Humanity has long sought the ability to live forever. Even though the idea of immortality may be a fantasy, there are several ways to uncover the secret to living the longest and healthiest life. This eBook, "The Secrets to Eternal Youth," will examine the science of aging, the importance of diet, exercise, and movement, stress management, mental health, sleep, and rest, as well as lifestyle decisions that support youth.

Chapter 1: The Science of Aging

In this chapter, readers will learn more about how the body is affected by aging naturally. They will investigate how genetics, environment, and lifestyle affect aging as well as the effects of inflammation and free radicals. In this chapter, readers will additionally stumble upon advice on how to delay aging.

Chapter 2: The Power of Nutrition

It is impossible to overestimate the value of healthy eating for a long life. The greatest foods to eat for good health and anti-aging advantages will be covered in this chapter, along with nutrients and supplements that support youth. The recommendations for food preparation and planning are also provided for the readers.

Chapter 3: Exercise and Movement

Regular exercise is vital to living a longer, healthier life. In this chapter, readers will learn about the different types of exercise and their benefits, as well as how to develop an exercise routine that fits their lifestyle. Tips for staying active and moving throughout the day will also be provided.

Chapter 4: Managing Stress and Mental Health

Stress and mental health can impact the aging process. This chapter will explore strategies for managing stress and anxiety, techniques for promoting relaxation and mindfulness, and the importance of social connections and support.

Chapter 5: Sleep and Rest

For lifespan and good health, sleep is essential. This chapter teaches readers how to get better sleep, the health advantages of relaxation and rest, and how to establish a nightly routine for restful sleep.

Chapter 6: Lifestyle Choices for Eternal Youth

Alcohol, drugs, and smoking are some substances that can slow down aging. This chapter will offer advice on how to take care of your skin, delay the aging process, stop smoking, and consume less alcohol. There will also be discussion of other lifestyle options that support adolescents.

Conclusion:

In conclusion, the reader will be reminded of the important ideas covered in the eBook and inspired to put the advise into practice. final observations on the quest.

Chapter 1

The Science of Aging

Understanding How the Body Ages

Aging is a natural and inevitable process that affects every living organism, including humans. It is characterized by a gradual decline in physiological functions, which can lead to a range of health problems, such as cardiovascular diseases, cancer, and neurodegenerative disorders. In recent years, there has been a growing interest in the science of aging, as researchers try to unravel the mechanisms underlying this complex process. In this chapter, we will explore how the body ages and the factors that contribute to this process.

- **Cellular Aging:** At the cellular level, aging is marked by a gradual accumulation of damage to DNA, proteins, and other cellular structures. This damage can be caused by a variety of factors, including oxidative stress, inflammation, and exposure to environmental toxins. Over time, this damage can impair cellular function, leading to a decline in tissue and organ function.

- **Telomere Shortening:** One of the most widely studied mechanisms of cellular aging is telomere shortening. Telomeres are the protective caps at the end of chromosomes that gradually shorten with each cell division. Once they become too short, cells can no longer divide and may enter a state of senescence or programmed cell death.

This process has been implicated in a range of age-related diseases, including cancer and Alzheimer's disease.

- **Epigenetic Changes:** In addition to cellular damage and telomere shortening, aging is also associated with epigenetic changes. Epigenetic modifications are chemical tags that attach to DNA and regulate gene expression. With age, these tags can become disrupted, leading to changes in gene expression patterns and altered cellular function. This can contribute to a range of age-related diseases, including cardiovascular disease and metabolic disorders.

- **Inflammation:** Another key factor in the aging process is chronic inflammation. Inflammation is a natural response to injury or infection, but it can become chronic and contribute to a range of age-related diseases, including cancer, heart disease, and neurodegenerative disorders. This chronic inflammation is thought to be driven by a variety of factors, including cellular damage, changes in the gut microbiome, and the accumulation of senescent cells.

- **Hormonal Changes:** Finally, hormonal changes also play a role in the aging process. As we age, levels of hormones such as estrogen, testosterone, and growth hormone decline, which can contribute to a range of age-related health problems, including osteoporosis, muscle loss, and cognitive decline. Hormonal changes may also contribute to the development of age-related diseases such as breast cancer and prostate cancer.

Understanding The Role Of Genetics, Environment, And Lifestyle

Aging is a complex process that is influenced by a wide range of factors, including genetics, environment, and lifestyle. In this chapter, we will delve into the science behind aging and explore how these different factors contribute to the aging process.

- **Genetics**

One of the most significant factors that influence aging is genetics. Our genes determine many of our physical and biological traits, including how our bodies age. Some people are genetically predisposed to age more slowly or to be more resistant to age-related diseases, while others may be more susceptible to the effects of aging.

Research has shown that genetic factors account for approximately 25% of the variation in human lifespan. There are several genes that have been linked to aging and age-related diseases, including the FOXO3A gene, which has been associated with longevity, and the APOE gene, which is linked to Alzheimer's disease.

However, genetics are not the only factor that influences aging. Our environment and lifestyle also play a crucial role.

- **Environment**

Environmental factors such as pollution, toxins, and exposure to the sun can all contribute to aging. Exposure to UV radiation from the sun, for example, can damage our skin and lead to wrinkles, age spots, and other signs of aging.

Pollution and toxins in the air and water can also contribute to the aging process by damaging our cells and DNA. This can lead to an increased risk of age-related diseases such as cancer, heart disease, and Alzheimer's disease.

Additionally, our environment can also influence the expression of our genes. Epigenetics, which refers to changes in gene expression that are not caused by changes to the underlying DNA sequence, can be influenced by environmental factors such as diet, stress, and exercise.

- **Lifestyle**

Our lifestyle choices also play a significant role in the aging process. Unhealthy habits such as smoking, excessive alcohol consumption, and a sedentary lifestyle can all accelerate the aging process and increase the risk of age-related diseases.

On the other hand, healthy lifestyle choices such as regular exercise, a balanced diet, and stress management techniques can help slow the aging process and reduce the risk of age-related diseases.

Research has shown that regular exercise can help improve cardiovascular health, maintain muscle mass, and improve cognitive function in older adults. A healthy diet that is rich in fruits, vegetables, whole grains, and lean protein can help reduce inflammation, improve gut health, and provide essential nutrients that support healthy aging.

Stress management techniques such as meditation, yoga, and deep breathing can also help reduce the impact of stress on the body, which can contribute to aging and age-related diseases.

The Impact Of Free Radicals And Inflammation On Aging

Aging is a complex process influenced by a wide range of factors. While genetics play a role, environmental factors, lifestyle choices, and cellular damage are also major contributors to the aging process. One of the key factors that contribute to aging is the accumulation of free radicals and inflammation in the body.

Free radicals are unstable molecules that are formed as a result of normal cellular metabolism, exposure to environmental toxins, and other stressors. These molecules can damage DNA, proteins, and lipids in the body, leading to cellular dysfunction and aging. In addition, free radicals can cause inflammation in the body, which is a natural response to injury or infection. However, chronic inflammation can lead to tissue damage and accelerate the aging process.

One of the primary mechanisms by which free radicals and inflammation contribute to aging is through damage to mitochondria. Mitochondria are the powerhouses of the cell and are responsible for producing energy. However, they are also highly susceptible to damage by free radicals. As a result, mitochondrial dysfunction can occur, leading to decreased energy production and an increase in oxidative stress.

In addition to damaging mitochondria, free radicals and inflammation can also contribute to the development of age-related diseases. For example, chronic inflammation has been linked to the development of cardiovascular disease, Alzheimer's disease, and cancer. Free radicals have also been linked to cancer development, as well as other age-related diseases.

Fortunately, there are several ways to reduce the impact of free radicals and inflammation on the aging process. One of the most effective ways is through diet. Antioxidants, which are found in fruits, vegetables, and other plant-based foods, can neutralize free radicals and reduce oxidative stress in the body. Additionally, consuming a diet that is rich in omega-3 fatty acids, such as those found in fatty fish, can help reduce inflammation in the body.

Regular exercise is also important for reducing the impact of free radicals and inflammation on the aging process. Exercise can help reduce oxidative stress in the body while also reducing inflammation. In addition, regular exercise can improve mitochondrial function, which can help increase energy production and reduce the impact of aging on the body.

How to Slow Down the Aging Process

As we discussed in the previous chapter, aging is a natural process that occurs in all living organisms. However, recent research has shown that there are ways to slow down this process and extend our lifespan. In this chapter, we will discuss some of the most effective strategies to slow down aging and promote longevity.

- **Exercise Regularly**

Regular exercise is one of the most effective ways to slow down the aging process. Exercise helps to maintain muscle mass and bone density, which can decline with age. It also helps to improve cardiovascular health, which can reduce the risk of age-related diseases such as heart disease and stroke. Additionally, exercise has been shown to improve cognitive function, which can help prevent age-related cognitive decline.

- **Eat a Healthy Diet**

Eating a healthy diet is another key factor in slowing down the aging process. A diet rich in fruits, vegetables, whole grains, and lean proteins can provide the body with the nutrients it needs to function at its best. In contrast, a diet high in processed foods, saturated fats, and sugar can contribute to inflammation and oxidative stress, both of which can accelerate aging.

- **Manage Stress**

Chronic stress has been shown to accelerate the aging process. It can contribute to inflammation, oxidative stress, and other processes that can damage cells and tissues. To manage stress, it is important to develop healthy coping mechanisms such as exercise, meditation, or spending time in nature. Additionally, practicing mindfulness and seeking support from friends and family can also help reduce stress levels.

- **Get Enough Sleep**

Getting enough sleep is essential for overall health and wellbeing. It is during sleep that the body repairs and regenerates cells and tissues. Chronic sleep deprivation has been linked to a range of health problems, including accelerated aging. To promote healthy sleep, it is important to maintain a regular sleep schedule, avoid caffeine and alcohol before bedtime, and create a relaxing sleep environment.

- **Protect Your Skin from the Sun**

Exposure to the sun's ultraviolet (UV) rays can damage the skin and accelerate the aging process. To protect your skin from the sun, it is important to wear sunscreen with at least SPF 30, wear protective clothing, and seek shade during the hottest part of the day.

- **Quit Smoking**

Smoking is one of the most significant contributors to premature aging. It can damage the skin, lungs, and other organs, and increase the risk of age-related diseases such as cancer and heart disease. Quitting smoking can help reduce the risk of these diseases and promote overall health and wellbeing.

Chapter 2

The Power of Nutrition

The importance of proper nutrition for longevity

Having a nutritious diet is essential for living a long and active life. Maintaining good health and avoiding chronic diseases that might shorten our lives depend on eating a balanced diet that contains all the required elements.

Research shows that the standard of nutrition and life expectancy are directly correlated. According to a Harvard University study, people who eat a healthy diet rich in whole grains, fruits, vegetables, nuts, and fish are less likely to die from any cause, including cancer and cardiovascular disease.

According to a second study, a Mediterranean diet rich in fruits, vegetables, wholegrains, legumes, and healthy fats has been associated with an increased lifespan. This report was also published in the Journal of the American Medical Association. According to the research, people who follow a Mediterranean-style diet have a lower risk of dying from cancer, heart disease, and other chronic diseases.

Nutrition can reduce the risk of developing chronic diseases while also delaying aging. A study by the National Institute of Aging has shown that animals can live as long as 50% longer if they eat a diet with little or no calorie content, but plenty of nutrients. It follows that if individuals eat fewer calories, but still receive all of the nutrients they need, they may live longer.

Nutrients for Longevity

So, in order to promote longevity, what nutrients should we be focusing on? Let's take a look at some key nutrients that can prolong your life and help you be more healthy:

- **Antioxidants:** Antioxidants protect cells against the damage caused by free radicals, which may lead to chronic disease and premature ageing. These foods contain a significant amount of antioxidants include berries, chocolate, nuts and green leafy vegetables.

- **Omega-3 Fatty Acids:** It has been shown that the important fatty acids are associated with reduced inflammation, improved heart health and protection from cognitive decline. A high level of Omega-3 fatty acid is found in fish, flaxseeds, chia seeds, and walnuts.

- **Fiber:** In order to maintain good gut microflora, which is essential for maintaining general health and longevity, fiber plays an important role. Foods with high fiber content are fruits, vegetables, grain products and legumes.

- **Vitamins and minerals:** To maintain optimal health and prevent lifelong illnesses, all essential vitamins and minerals need to be obtained. Fruits, vegetables, whole grains, nuts and seeds are foods that have a high content of vitamins and minerals.

Foods to Eat for Optimal Health and Anti-Aging Benefits

In the previous chapter, we discussed the power of nutrition and how it can help us live longer and healthier lives. Now, we'll look at the foods that can deliver optimal health and anti-aging benefits to us.

- **Berries**

The berries contain antioxidants that help fight off free radicals in the body, which can cause cellular damage and accelerate aging. There are a lot of great choices, including blueberries, raspberries, blackberries, and strawberries.

- **Leafy Greens**

The vitamins and minerals needed for good health are found in leafy greens such as spinach, kale, or collard greens. They're also rich in antioxidants that are capable of preventing damage to our cells.

- **Fatty Fish**

Omega 3 fatty acids, which have been shown to reduce inflammation and reduce the risk of chronic diseases such as heart disease and diabetes, are found in fish such as salmon, mackerel, and sardines.

- **Nuts and Seeds**

There are nutrients such as healthy fats, proteins, and fibers in nuts and seeds. They're also filled with antioxidants and other substances that can guard against damage to our cells.

- **Whole Grains**

Fiber, which can help regulate blood sugar levels and promote digestive health, is present in whole grains such as brown rice, quinoa, and wholewheat bread. They're also rich in vitamins and minerals that are essential for good health.

- **Fermented Foods**

Fermented foods such as yogurt, kefir, sauerkraut, and kimchi contain probiotics, which are beneficial bacteria that can promote digestive health and boost our immune system.

- **Colorful Fruits and Vegetables**

vitamins and minerals, as well as antioxidants that can protect cells from damage, are abundant in colorful fruits and vegetables such as carrots, sweet potatoes, tomatoes, and bell peppers.

- **Herbs and Spices**

There are compounds in herbs and spices, such as turmeric, ginger, garlic and cinnamon has the ability to reduce inflammation and protect against oxidative damage.

Note: The key to optimum health and the benefits of antiaging is a diet rich in pure, nutrient-dense foods. In addition, we can feed our bodies with the nutrients and antioxidants that are needed to sustain longevity and vitality by incorporating these foods into our diet.

Nutrients and Supplements That Promote Youthfulness

Proper food intake is one of the main factors in maintaining a youthful and healthy body. Food is an essential component in our body's building blocks for every cell, and a proper balance of nutrients can help protect us from diseases, promote healthy aging, and maintain the best functioning of our bodies. Some of the main nutrients and supplements that can help maintain youth and vitality will be explored in this chapter.

Antioxidants

Antioxidant vitamins are one of the main nutrients for promoting youthfulness. These substances prevent free radicals in the body that can lead to cellular damage, contributing to aging and disease. The following are some of the most promising sources of antioxidants:

- **Fruits and vegetables:** Antioxidant-rich fruits and vegetables include dark leafy greens, berries, citrus fruits, and cruciferous vegetables such as broccoli and kale.

- **Nuts and Seeds:** There are a lot of sources of antioxidants in nuts and seeds, such as almonds, walnuts, pumpkin, and sunflower seeds.

- **Spices:** All spices are rich in antioxidants and have been shown to have anti inflammatory properties, for example, turmeric, ginger, cinnamon, or cloves.

It's also a good idea to add antioxidants, in particular when you find it difficult to eat too much of them. A few of the most frequently used antioxidant supplements are as follows:

- **Vitamin C:** For collagen synthesis and skin health, this potent antioxidant is essential.

- **Vitamin E:** Another important antioxidant, vitamin E is helpful in protecting against oxidative stress and may help mitigate the risk of CVDs.

- **Coenzyme Q10 (CoQ10):** Is important to the production of cell energy, and protection from oxidative damage can also be provided by this antioxidant.

Omega-3 Fatty Acids

The form of fat known as omega-3 polyunsaturated fatty acids is indispensable for the brain, heart, and overall state of health. Maintaining youthful, healthy skin, hair, and nails is also influenced by these good fats. The following are some of the most significant sources of omega-3 fatty acids:

- Fish with high levels of Omega-3 fatty acids like salmon, mackerel, and sardines. Chia and flaxseeds are great sources of omega-3 fatty acids in vegan diets.

- Chia seeds and flax seeds are very good sources of omega-3 fatty acids for vegetarians.

- Walnuts are also a good source of omega-3 fatty acids.

You may be considering using an omega-3 supplement if you do not eat enough of these foods. Look for supplements that contain both EPA and DHA, two types of omega-3 fatty acids that have a particularly beneficial effect on health.

Collagen

Collagen is a protein essential to maintaining healthy skin, hair, nails, and joints. We naturally lose collagen production in our bodies as we get older, which can lead to wrinkles, aging skin, and other problems with joints. Fortunately, it is possible to strengthen these areas' youthful vitality by adding collagen.

There are many different forms of collagen supplements available, such as powders, capsules, and drinks. For the best skin health, you should check for supplements containing type 1 collagen, which is most abundant in your body and is of particular importance.

Vitamin D

For bone health, immune function, and overall healthy living, vitamin D is an essential nutrient. This nutrient is also important for maintaining healthy, youthful skin and may help prevent skin aging due to sun exposure.

The best source of vitamin D is sunlight, but many people don't get enough sun exposure to meet their needs. In these cases, supplementation may be necessary. Look for vitamin D3 supplements, which are more effective at raising vitamin D levels than other forms of the nutrient.

Tips for Meal Planning and Preparation

Now that we understand the importance of nutrition in our quest for eternal youth, let's dive deeper into how we can plan and prepare our meals to optimize our health.

- **Start with a balanced plate.**

A balanced plate should consist of 50% non-starchy vegetables, 25% lean protein, and 25% complex carbohydrates. This will help you meet your daily nutrient requirements while keeping you full and satisfied.

- **Plan your meals ahead of time.**

Planning your meals ahead of time can save you time, money, and stress. You can create a weekly meal plan and grocery list, and prepare your meals in advance. This way, you'll always have healthy options on hand and won't be tempted to reach for junk food.

- **Batch Cook**

Batch cooking is a great way to save time and ensure you have healthy meals available when you need them. Cook large batches of grains, proteins, and vegetables and store them in separate containers in the fridge or freezer. Then, when you're ready to eat, you can mix and match these components to create a variety of meals.

- **Use herbs and spices.**

Herbs and spices not only add flavor to your meals, but they also have many health benefits. For example, turmeric is anti-inflammatory, garlic is antibacterial, and ginger aids in digestion. Experiment with different herbs and spices to add flavor and nutrition to your meals.

- **Choose whole foods.**

Whole foods, such as fruits, vegetables, whole grains, and lean proteins, are packed with nutrients that are essential for good health. They also tend to be more filling and satisfying than processed foods. Aim to fill your plate with whole foods and limit your intake of processed and packaged foods.

- **Stay hydrated.**

Staying hydrated is essential for good health. Aim to drink at least eight glasses of water per day, and more if you're active or live in a hot climate. You can also hydrate with herbal teas, coconut water, and fresh juices.

- **Listen to your body.**

Finally, it's important to listen to your body and eat intuitively. Pay attention to how your body feels after you eat certain foods, and adjust your diet accordingly. If you feel bloated or sluggish after eating a certain food, it may be best to avoid it in the future.
By following these tips for meal planning and preparation, you can ensure that you're fueling your body with the nutrients it needs to thrive. Remember, the key to eternal youth is not just living a long life but a healthy and fulfilling one.

Chapter 3

Exercise and Movement

In Chapter 2, we discussed the power of nutrition and its impact on living a longer, healthier life. In this chapter, we will explore the benefits of exercise and the different types of exercise that can help you achieve your health goals.

The Benefits of Exercise for a Longer, Healthier Life

Exercise is a crucial component of a healthy lifestyle, and the benefits of exercise are numerous. Regular physical activity can help you:

- **Improve cardiovascular health:** Exercise can help lower blood pressure, reduce the risk of heart disease and stroke, and improve blood circulation.

- **Maintain a healthy weight:** Exercise can help you burn calories, maintain muscle mass, and improve your metabolism, all of which contribute to a healthy weight.

- **Reduce the risk of chronic diseases:** Exercise can reduce the risk of developing chronic diseases such as type 2 diabetes, some forms of cancer, and osteoporosis.

- **Improve mental health:** Exercise has been shown to reduce symptoms of depression and anxiety and improve overall mood.

- **Increase longevity:** Regular exercise has been linked to a longer life expectancy and a lower risk of premature death.

Different Types of Exercise and Their Benefits

There are several different types of exercise, each with its own unique benefits. Some of the most popular types of exercise include:

- **Aerobic exercise:** Aerobic exercise, also known as cardio, is any exercise that increases your heart rate and breathing, such as running, cycling, or swimming. Aerobic exercise is great for improving cardiovascular health, burning calories, and reducing the risk of chronic diseases.

- **Strength training:** Strength training involves using resistance, such as weights or resistance bands, to build muscle and improve strength. Strength training is important for maintaining muscle mass, improving metabolism, and reducing the risk of injury.

- **Flexibility training:** Flexibility training, such as yoga or stretching, improves joint mobility and range of motion. It can also help reduce the risk of injury and improve posture.

- **High-intensity interval training (HIIT):** HIIT involves short bursts of intense exercise followed by periods of rest or lower-intensity exercise. It can be a great way to burn calories, improve cardiovascular health, and increase metabolism.

- **Balance training:** Balance training, such as yoga or tai chi, improves balance and coordination, which can reduce the risk of falls and improve overall mobility.

It's important to incorporate a variety of different types of exercise into your routine to achieve maximum benefits. For example, combining aerobic exercise with strength training and flexibility training can help you achieve overall fitness and improve your health and longevity.

How to develop an exercise routine that fits your lifestyle

Developing an exercise routine that fits your lifestyle is essential to maintaining consistency and achieving your health goals. Here are some steps you can take to develop an exercise routine that works for you:

- **Assess your current fitness level:** Before starting any exercise routine, it's important to assess your current fitness level. This will help you determine what types of exercises are appropriate for you and how much you should be doing. If you're unsure about your fitness level, consider consulting with a personal trainer or healthcare professional.

- **Set realistic goals:** It's important to set realistic goals that are achievable for your fitness level and lifestyle. Whether you want to lose weight, build muscle, or simply improve your overall health, setting achievable goals will help you stay motivated and focused.

- **Choose activities you enjoy**: One of the keys to developing an exercise routine that you'll stick to is choosing activities that you enjoy. Whether it's running, yoga, swimming, or weightlifting, finding an activity that you enjoy will make it easier to stay committed and consistent.

- **Create a schedule:** Creating a schedule for your exercise routine can help you stay on track and ensure that you're making time for physical activity. Consider scheduling your workouts at the same time each day or week to establish a routine.

- **Make it social:** Exercising with a friend or joining a fitness class can make physical activity more enjoyable and keep you motivated. Consider finding a workout buddy or joining a local fitness group to help you stay on track.

Tips for staying active and moving throughout the day

In addition to structured exercise, it's important to stay active and move throughout the day. Here are some tips for incorporating physical activity into your daily routine:

- **Take breaks:** If you work at a desk job, it's important to take breaks throughout the day to stand up, stretch, and move around. Consider setting a timer to remind you to take a break every hour or so.

- **Walk more:** Walking is an easy and low-impact way to stay active throughout the day. Consider walking to work or taking a stroll during your lunch break.

- **Use the stairs:** Instead of taking the elevator or escalator, opt for the stairs whenever possible. This can help increase your heart rate and burn some extra calories.

Find ways to incorporate movement into your daily tasks: Whether it's doing squats while brushing your teeth or taking a walk during a phone call, finding ways to incorporate movement into your daily tasks can help increase your overall physical activity.

Stay active with hobbies: Hobbies like gardening, dancing, or playing a sport can provide a fun and enjoyable way to stay active and move your body.

Chapter 4

Managing Stress and Mental Health

In this chapter, we will explore the impact of stress and mental health on the aging process. Stress is a natural part of life, but when it becomes chronic and unmanaged, it can have detrimental effects on our physical and mental well-being. It is important to understand how stress affects the body and mind and to develop strategies for managing stress and anxiety in order to live a longer, healthier life.

How stress and mental health impact the aging process

Stress and mental health can have a significant impact on the aging process. Chronic stress can lead to a variety of health problems, including high blood pressure, heart disease, diabetes, and depression. These conditions can, in turn, accelerate the aging process, leading to a shorter lifespan and a lower quality of life.

Mental health is also closely linked to the aging process. Depression, anxiety, and other mental health disorders can have physical effects on the body, such as increased inflammation, oxidative stress, and cellular aging. These effects can contribute to the development of chronic diseases and other age-related health problems.

Strategies for managing stress and anxiety

Fortunately, there are a variety of strategies that can help manage stress and anxiety and promote mental health. Here are some effective strategies to consider:

- **Exercise:** Regular exercise is one of the best ways to manage stress and promote mental health. Exercise releases endorphins, which are natural mood boosters, and can also help reduce inflammation and oxidative stress in the body. Aim for at least 30 minutes of moderate exercise most days of the week.

- **Mindfulness meditation:** Mindfulness meditation is a powerful tool for managing stress and anxiety. It involves focusing your attention on the present moment and accepting your thoughts and feelings without judgment. Research has shown that regular mindfulness meditation can reduce symptoms of anxiety and depression and even slow cellular aging.

- **Yoga:** Yoga is another effective way to manage stress and anxiety. It combines physical movement with mindfulness meditation and can help reduce inflammation, lower blood pressure, and improve sleep quality.

- **Social support:** Social support is essential for good mental health. Spending time with loved ones, participating in group activities, and seeking professional counseling can all help reduce stress and improve overall well-being.

- **Sleep hygiene:** Good sleep is essential for managing stress and promoting mental health. Aim for 7-9 hours of sleep per night and practice good sleep hygiene habits, such as avoiding screens before bedtime, keeping your bedroom dark and quiet, and avoiding caffeine and alcohol in the evening.

The importance of social connections and support

- **Reduce loneliness and isolation**: Loneliness and isolation can have a negative impact on mental health. Maintaining social connections can help reduce feelings of loneliness and isolation.

- **Increase self-esteem:** Social connections can help boost self-esteem and self-worth. Having a support system can help you feel valued and loved.

- **Provide emotional support:** Social connections can provide emotional support during difficult times. Having someone to talk to and share your experiences with can be invaluable.

Improve overall health: Social connections have been shown to improve overall health and longevity. People with strong social connections tend to have better physical and mental health.

- **Expand your social circle:** Don't be afraid to branch out and meet new people. Join a club or group that interests you, or take a class to learn a new skill. You never know who you might meet or how they could impact your life.

In conclusion, managing stress and mental health is an essential part of living a long, healthy life. Incorporating relaxation and mindfulness techniques into your daily routine and maintaining social connections and support can help reduce stress, improve mental health, and increase overall well-being. By taking care of your mental health, you are also taking care of your physical health, so make it a priority.

Chapter 5
Sleep and Rest

Sleep is an essential component of a healthy lifestyle and is vital to maintaining good physical and mental health. It plays a crucial role in regulating the body's functions, including metabolism, the immune system, and hormone production. Adequate sleep is associated with a reduced risk of chronic diseases such as diabetes, heart disease, and obesity, and it is also linked to improved cognitive function, emotional well-being, and overall quality of life. In this chapter, we will explore the critical role of sleep and rest in maintaining eternal youth and how to optimize your sleep quality.

The Role of Sleep in Overall Health and Longevity

Sleep is a restorative process that helps the body repair and rejuvenate itself. During sleep, the body repairs damaged tissues, consolidates memories, and removes toxins from the brain. Lack of sleep or poor quality sleep can lead to a range of health problems, including chronic fatigue, weight gain, a weakened immune system, and an increased risk of heart disease, stroke, and diabetes.

Recent studies have shown that sleep plays a vital role in regulating the body's biological clock, which influences the timing of various physiological processes. Disruptions to the body's internal clock, such as those caused by shift work, can have negative effects on health, including an increased risk of cancer.

Tips for Improving Sleep Quality

There are several strategies you can use to improve the quality of your sleep. These include:

- **Establish a regular sleep schedule:** Go to bed and wake up at the same time every day, even on weekends.

- **Create a relaxing sleep environment:** Keep your bedroom cool, dark, and quiet, and avoid using electronics in bed.

- **Reduce caffeine and alcohol intake:** Avoid caffeine and alcohol in the evening, as they can disrupt sleep.

- **Practice relaxation techniques:** Try deep breathing, meditation, or yoga to help relax your mind and body before bed.

- **Get regular exercise:** Exercise during the day can help improve sleep quality, but avoid intense exercise close to bedtime.

The Benefits of Rest and Relaxation for the Body and Mind

Rest and relaxation are essential components of maintaining good health and well-being. They help reduce stress, lower blood pressure, and improve mood. In addition, rest and relaxation can also improve cognitive function, memory, and creativity.

Rest and relaxation can take many forms, including spending time in nature, taking a warm bath, reading a book, or listening to music. It's essential to make time for rest and relaxation in your daily routine, even if it's just for a few minutes each day.

How to Create a Bedtime Routine for Optimal Rest

Creating a bedtime routine can help signal to your body that it's time to sleep. Here are some steps you can take to create a bedtime routine for optimal rest:

Set a regular bedtime and wake-up time.

- **Wind down before bed:** Avoid using electronic devices and instead read a book, take a bath, or listen to relaxing music.

- **Create a relaxing sleep environment:** Keep your bedroom cool, dark, and quiet.

- **Practice relaxation techniques:** Try deep breathing, meditation, or yoga to help relax your mind and body.

- **Avoid stimulants:** Avoid caffeine, alcohol, and nicotine before bedtime, as they can interfere with sleep.

In conclusion, sleep and rest are essential components of maintaining good health and well-being. By making sleep and rest a priority in your daily routine, you can unlock the secrets to eternal youth and live your longest, healthiest life. Use the tips and strategies outlined in this chapter to optimize your sleep quality and make rest and relaxation a regular part of your life.

Chapter 6

Lifestyle Choices for Eternal Youth

In this chapter, we'll delve into some of the most important lifestyle choices that can help you maintain your youthfulness and live a longer, healthier life. We'll focus on three key areas: quitting smoking and reducing alcohol intake; protecting your skin and preventing premature aging; and other lifestyle choices that promote youthfulness.

Tips for Quitting Smoking and Reducing Alcohol Intake

Smoking and excessive alcohol consumption are two of the most significant factors that can accelerate the aging process and increase the risk of developing serious health problems. If you're a smoker or a heavy drinker, quitting or reducing your intake can be one of the most important steps you can take to improve your overall health and well-being. Here are some tips to help you get started:

- **Make a plan:** Quitting smoking or reducing your alcohol intake can be a challenging process, so it's important to have a plan in place. Set a specific date to quit or start reducing your intake, and create a plan that includes strategies to help you manage cravings and cope with stress.

- **Seek support:** Don't be afraid to ask for help from friends, family members, or a healthcare professional. Support from others can be crucial in helping you stick to your plan and achieve your goals.

- **Find alternatives:** If you're struggling with cravings or the urge to drink or smoke, try to find alternative ways to cope. Exercise, meditation, or hobbies like reading or painting can be great ways to distract yourself and manage stress.

- **Be patient:** Quitting smoking or reducing your alcohol intake can take time, and it's important to be patient with yourself. Remember that setbacks are normal, and it's okay to ask for help if you need it.

How to Protect Your Skin and Prevent Premature Aging

Protecting your skin is essential for maintaining your youthfulness and preventing premature aging. Exposure to the sun's UV rays, pollution, and other environmental factors can damage your skin and accelerate the aging process. Here are some tips to help you protect your skin:

- **Wear sunscreen**: Sunscreen is essential for protecting your skin from the sun's harmful UV rays. Choose a broad-spectrum sunscreen with an SPF of at least 30, and apply it regularly throughout the day.

- **Cover up:** If you're going to be spending time in the sun, wear protective clothing like a hat, sunglasses, and long sleeves.

- **Avoid smoking:** Smoking can damage your skin and accelerate the aging process. If you're a smoker, quitting can help improve the appearance of your skin and reduce the risk of developing wrinkles and other signs of aging.

- **Stay hydrated:** Drinking plenty of water can help keep your skin hydrated and prevent dryness and wrinkles.

Conclusion

Congratulations on completing this new book "The Secrets to Eternal Youth: Uncovering the Hidden Path To Living Your Longest, Healthiest Life"! This comprehensive guide to living a longer, healthier life is an excellent resource for anyone looking to improve their overall well-being.

A recap of key points

Throughout the book, you have provided readers with valuable insights and practical tips for achieving eternal youth. You have emphasized the importance of maintaining a healthy lifestyle by eating a balanced diet, engaging in regular physical activity, getting enough sleep, and managing stress. Additionally, you have highlighted the importance of maintaining strong social connections, pursuing hobbies, and engaging in cognitive activities to keep the mind sharp.

Encouragement to implement the advice in daily life

While the pursuit of eternal youth may seem daunting, it's important to remember that every small step towards a healthier lifestyle counts. Implementing the advice provided in this book may seem challenging at first, but it's crucial to take it one day at a time and gradually incorporate healthy habits into your daily routine. Whether it's swapping out processed foods for whole, nutrient-dense options or taking a daily walk around the neighborhood, every effort towards a healthier lifestyle is a step in the right direction.

Final thoughts on the pursuit of eternal youth

In the end, it's essential to remember that the pursuit of eternal youth is not about looking younger or defying the aging process entirely. Instead, it's about improving the quality of life and feeling your best at every age. By following the advice outlined in this book, you'll be able to achieve a healthier, happier, and more fulfilling life. Remember that the journey towards eternal youth is a lifelong process, and it's never too late to start making positive changes in your life. With dedication, consistency, and a positive attitude, you can achieve the longevity and vitality you deserve.